Christ Healing in the Parish

by
Michael Botting
Joint Director of Training, Diocese of Chester

GROVE BOOKS LIMITED
Bramcote   Nottingham   NG9 3DS

CONTENTS

		Page
	Preface	3
1.	Introduction	5
2.	Miraculous Healing in the Bible	7
3.	Miraculous Healing Today	12
4.	Christian Healing Today	15
5.	Conclusion	24
6.	Bibliography	25

Copyright Michael Botting 1976, 1977, 1985 and 1992

ACKNOWLEDGEMENTS

I am especially indebted to the Rev. Dr. John Stott for an address given at St. George's, Leeds, on the subject of miraculous healing before an audience of doctors and nurses. Also my thanks go to Dr. and Mrs. Michael Flowers and to the Rev. Nicholas Sagovsky for reading the original manuscript and making a number of very helpful suggestions. Finally I must add my gratitude to Elaine Naish (nee Phillips) for deciphering my handwriting and typing and retyping the manuscript.

Michael Botting
August 1992

THE COVER PICTURE
is by Roy Dean

First Edition February 1976
Second Edition September 1977
Third Edition May 1985
Fourth Edition (by Grove Books Limited) October 1992
ISSN 0305-3067
ISBN 1 85174 225 5

PREFACE

'If I discovered a lump', my wife explained to some Christian friends over tea, 'I should not attempt to hide what the trouble might be and I should expect laying-on-of-hands or anointing.' Within less than 24 hours of those remarks being made a lump had been discovered, the doctor seen, and an appointment with a specialist at the Royal Marsden Hospital arranged. I had been away on a conference where a number of things had happened that in various ways had prepared me for the news. So a few months before removing to a new sphere of ministry I had to come to terms with the possibility that my wife might have to undergo major surgery.

As soon as the situation had been explained we contacted two personal friends, an Anglican clergyman and his wife, whom we knew to exercise a ministry of healing in their parish. They gladly came over on the following Saturday and several of us gathered round my wife while hands were laid on her and prayer offered.

Quite remarkably, a bed in the hospital was available on the Monday, only a week after the lump had first been discovered. On the Tuesday I personally experienced a tremendous sense of peace, so much so that a friend at a Deanery Chapter Meeting that morning commented upon it. The operation took place and was perhaps a little worse than had originally been expected. But my wife was allowed out of hospital in nine days.

The eight-week radium treatment not only fitted exactly between our pre-arranged holidays but on the very first day of treatment my wife experienced an inner healing and warmth spread throughout her body. The medical staff were astonished that she responded so well, especially with her fair skin. Over 20 years since the operation have brought no after-effects. She was discharged by the medical profession over 14 years ago.

Why it was necessary for the lump at all is all part of the problem of pain and disease which is the lot of this fallen world. However in this incident we were aware of the Lord's 'healing hand', not just in the skill given to surgeon, doctors and nurses, but in the ministry of Christian friends as well as in the Lord's ordering of circumstances. My wife has had an especial ministry to others finding themselves in similar circumstances to ours.

I recount this particular personal incident at the very beginning of this booklet so that readers may know (1) that I am not unfamiliar with some of the issues that surround the subject and (2) that the answer to prayers for healing may not be thought to by-pass the medical profession.

The first edition of this booklet appeared in 1976. At the time I expressed my hesitation to write on such a controversial subject, bearing in mind:
(1) We were living in the days of the so-called 'charismatic divide' in the church of Christ, part of the divide relating to charismatic emphasis on supernatural healing.
(2) The medical profession seemed divided on what part the miraculous played in healing, and I had no more medical knowledge than the average layman.
(3) The shelves of Christian bookshops were already loaded with books on healing.

Could I say anything that was new and biblically balanced? The answer seems clear from the fact that Grove Books continue to have sufficient requests each year to justify this fourth edition. Possibly, too, Mr. Archie McAdam, Consultant Surgeon of the Airedale General Hospital, continues to pass on copies to his cancer support group (for which purpose he sponsored the third edition in 1985). Then since the publication of the first edition the report *Gospel and Spirit* has been published, co-sponsored by the Church of England Evangelical Council and the Fountain Trust (now disbanded)[1], which has helped to close the 'charismatic divide'. But the evident pressure by charismatic groups and individuals on the late David Watson during the last year of his life as he struggled with terminal cancer, suggests there is still confusion on this subject. This is not just my opinion. Lots of people have quite independently expressed it to me after reading David's last (posthumous) book, *Fear no Evil* (Hodder 1984).

Then the very fact that I did write in the first place has meant that I have been invited to speak on healing in quite a few places, and the discussion that has followed has further concentrated and clarified my own thinking.

For the past decade John Wimber, the charismatic founding pastor of the Vineyard Christian Fellowship, has had a prominent ministry in Britain, but confess that I have not yet attended any of his meetings or those run by his team. I expect to remedy that omission shortly. However I have struggled with his book *Power Healing* (Hodder 1986) and much he writes is completely contrary to what I attempt to say in this booklet. The limitations of space prevent me from enlarging, except to mention three books directly related to this matter, namely: *HEALING: Fiction, Fantasy or Fact?* (Hodder) by Dr. David Lewis, *Signs and Wonders: The Wimber Phenomenon* (Daybreak) by John Gunstone and *The Question of HEALING SERVICES* (Daybreak) by John Richards, particularly chapter 3.

So that I may spare potential readers a wasted journey I will explain the general slant of the booklet. Imagine we are confronted with a person who is obviously not well, nor enjoying a state of physical, mental and social health—as Christians what can we do? There are three possibilities:

(1) We can say with total confidence that by applying spiritual ministrations such as prayer, laying on of hands, and anointing with oil, the patient should more or less immediately be cured and remain so, possibly with occasional repeated ministrations, until around seventy years of age when death will occur, because 'it is appointed for men to die...' (Heb. 9.27) and we can only expect to live about seventy years (Ps. 90.10). The Lord commissioned his disciples to heal the sick and all things are possible to those who have faith.

(2) Our patient can be told that the Lord has provided the world with food, but we still have to harvest it; likewise he has provided medical properties in the earth and doctors, so we should use them.

I suspect that no one really believes that either of these extremes is tenable: the first would make the medical profession unnecessary, and the second would deny the church any ministry of healing, so:

(3) There must be a middle way that is both biblical and true to actual experience. That is what this booklet examines.

[1] Now obtainable from Grove Books.

1. INTRODUCTION

The vital importance of the subject

This cannot be overstressed for several reasons:

(1) The Bible and especially the Gospels have a great deal of space devoted to miracles of healing—'Nearly one-fifth of the entire Gospels'.[1] The gift of healing is included amongst the gifts of the Spirit within the Body of Christ (1 Cor. 12.9).

(2) Christian compassion demands that the Church ministers to the sick both individually by visits from clergy and laity and corporately as a local expression of the Body of Christ.

(3) We are all likely to be ill at some time or other and therefore want to enjoy the full benefits of all God promises us in his Word.

(4) We do not want to raise the hopes of the sick and suffering beyond what is promised in Scripture. Without wishing to sound a discordant note, the fact of the matter is that we are all eventually to die, unless the Lord returns first—'it is appointed for men to die . . .' (Heb. 9.27).

All healing is of God

The God of nature and of means is also the God of grace and of miracle. Much healing therefore will be the direct result of natural causes. If this were not God's intention we need to ask why he created so much material with healing properties. As Ecclesiasticus 38.1-4 in the Apocrypha says, 'Hold the physician in honour, for he is essential to you, and God it was who established his profession. From God the doctor has his wisdom and the king provides for his sustenance. His knowledge makes the doctor distinguished, and gives him access to those in authority. God makes the earth yield healing herbs which the prudent man should not neglect.'

Paul Tournier also writes that in his experience technology and faith work together, 'Psychoanalysis explores the problems in order to bring them out into the daylight. Grace dissolves them without our ever knowing exactly how.'[2] Psychoanalysis may seem pretty godless at times but we must believe that it can be as much part of the divine activity as grace itself.

Francis MacNutt in his book *Healing* writes: 'Sometimes God works through nature and the skill of doctors; sometimes he works directly through prayer and sometimes through both, but always there should be co-operation, mutual respect and an admiration for the variety of ways in which God manifests his glory.'[3]

Because I believe that all healing is of God it may therefore seem a bit misleading to suggest that some is 'miraculous'. Nonetheless, I believe in the end that it is helpful to make such a distinction. I do so in the good company of Dr. Henry W. Frost whose book *Miraculous Healing* (Marshall, Morgan and Scott, 1951) I would particularly recommend.[4]

By the term 'miraculous' I simply mean healing instantaneously, without any apparent means and with some permanence. This definition is assumed in all that follows.

---

[1] Morton Kelsey *Healing and Christianity* (SCM) p.54.
[2] From *The Person Reborn* p.37—quoted in *Healing* by Francis MacNutt (Ave Maria Press) p.273.
[3] *Ibid.* p.274.
[4] Dr. D. Martyn Lloyd-Jones said of this book, 'It is easily and incomparably the best book I have ever read on this subject.'

The need for truth and honesty

On this crucial subject we must seek to the very best of our ability to be true to Scripture and modern medical science and also scrupulously accurate in our reporting. If we are otherwise we could end up by being positively cruel rather than compassionate. If at any point in what follows readers feel I have appeared a bit too negative then I would reply that I have been more concerned with what is true than what is an attractive, but nonetheless unjustified, optimism.

Medical scientists admit that their knowledge of the 'laws of nature' are still only limited and that sometimes cures occur for inexplicable reasons.

Many Anglican clergy to my knowledge used to receive news of quite astonishing healing conducted by an American pentecostal. One such healing involved the lengthening of a leg. A very well-known Anglican minister and a consultant in the National Health Service investigated this further and discovered that the case was not so simple as had been so widely reported. When these men attempted to enquire into further healings they were told that names and addresses were not being released. One of the cases of healing mentioned in one of the books in the bibliography has been followed up and it has been discovered that the present condition of the patient is by no means so glowing as the author of the book might lead us to expect. This naturally makes one suspect some of the other accounts described in the same book.[1]

A personal friend of mine had a very serious illness that was expected to prove fatal. Hands were laid on him and there was certainly a very remarkable degree of recovery, sufficient to enable him to return to his normal work and to do it with some competence. However if you met him you would be in no doubt at once that he is still a fairly disabled man. It was for that reason that I was disturbed by a letter of his to the editor of the *Church of England Newspaper* in which he stated: 'I believe that God is always willing to heal and that he does heal when we allow him to. I believe that this is what his word teaches.'

I leave my readers to make their own judgment, but I would imagine most people would assume the writer of that letter was enjoying a much greater degree of health than is still in fact the case. Total honesty is needed.

Christian healing cannot be separated from salvation

Salvation and 'wholeness' are practically interchangeable in Scripture. The Greek word 'sozo' is used to mean *both* 'save' *and* 'heal'. Jesus frequently spoke about the priority of the forgiveness of a sick person's sins before healing the body, as for example in Mark 2.3-12 (with parallels in Matthew 9 and Luke 5) of a paralytic who is brought before Jesus by four friends.

Lord Coggan, former Archbishop of Canterbury, makes the interesting comment, 'When Tyndale makes Christ say to Zacchaeus, "This day is *health* come to thy house" (where the Authorized Version says "salvation" —St. Luke 19.9 "soteria"), his translation spoke deeper then than he knew, and made luminous the deep interest of Christ, for true health is impossible apart from God.'[2]

---

[1] For a further instance see the detached footnote on p.24 below.
[2] F. D. Coggan *Convictions* (Hodder, 1975), pp.272-3.

2. MIRACULOUS HEALING IN THE BIBLE

(1) The Old Testament
Miraculous healing in the Old Testament is less frequent than is generally supposed and the few cases seem to be associated with two critical periods in Israel's history, namely the Exodus under Moses and the ministry of Elijah and Elisha. Moses prayed for his sister Miriam's healing from leprosy and set up the bronze serpent for the healing of serpent bite (Numbers 12.1-15 and 21.6-9). Both these early prophets cured children and Elisha was directly instrumental in the Syrian Commander Naaman's being cured of leprosy.

These healings were undoubtedly understood as special interventions of God and not his normal method of working. Direction for health, hygiene and sanitation is scattered throughout the Pentateuch, especially in Leviticus, to help the Israelites avoid disease and to instruct them what normal action they should take if illness should strike them.

These healings seem to have been understood as signs principally to authenticate the authority of the men who performed them. As the woman whose son Elijah cured said, 'Now I know that you are a man of God, and that the word of the Lord in your mouth is truth,' (1 Kings 17.24).

It is to be noted that the Egyptian magicians apparently performed miracles (Exodus 7.22). These may have been counterfeits or possibly initiated by occult forces. Whatever they were, God put a limit on them, for these sorcerers could not cope with the plague of boils (Exodus 9.11).

(2) The Gospels
Here we are primarily concerned with the healing ministry of Jesus. We are quite specifically told that John the Baptist did no miracles (John 10.41). Obviously in a booklet of this size we must be brief so we will make a number of general observations:

(i) *Jesus's healing ministry was extraordinarily extensive*
'Nearly one-fifth of the entire Gospels is devoted to Jesus' healing and the discussions occasioned by it' writes Morton Kelsey in his book *Healing and Christianity* and goes on to point out that 'except for miracles in general, that is by far the greatest emphasis given to any one kind of experience in the narrative.'[1]

Edmunds and Scorer in *Some Thoughts on Faith Healing*[2] write about the wide variety of diseases that Jesus dealt with, 'They would today be classified under several medical categories. They certainly included the blind, the maimed, the lame, the dumb, and those suffering from leprosy, fevers, menorrhagia, paralysis, kyphosis and epilepsy. In addition, the dead were restored to life. Exorcism of evil spirits was also performed.'

---
[1] *Healing and Christianity* (SCM) p.54.
[2] Tyndale Press p.19.

Apart from the case of the clay and spittle to which I make some reference below, Jesus did not use material means. The healings were normally immediate and complete, with no record of any relapses (though presumably all those cured would eventually have died—including those who had been restored to life). This accords with my definition of 'miraculous' healing mentioned in the Introduction on page 5.[1]

(ii) *Most of the conditions Jesus cured are still beyond the competence of medicine to cure.*
This is the view of Edmunds and Scorer writing in 1956.

(iii) *Jesus was not against the use of material means.*
He refers to the medicinal use of oil and wine in the parable of the Good Samaritan and uses clay made with spittle 'which was a popular remedy of the time for blindness (Mark 8.23, John 9.6) and deafness (Mark 7.32-35)' according to A. P. Waterson[2], who adds 'This may have been to aid the patient's faith or to demonstrate that God does not exclude the use of means, or both.' Jesus also said: 'Those who are well have no need of a physician, but those who are sick' (Matt. 9.12 and parallels), so he was not against the medical profession!

(iv) *Jesus helps clarify the relation of sin to sickness.*
It is generally accepted that suffering and disease is one of the results of human sin.[3] This would be generally confirmed by Jesus's whole attitude to physical and mental sickness which was one of anger. Dr. Coggan explains how when faced with a leper and with the death of Lazarus, the better way to describe Jesus's reaction would be to say he snorted like a horse. 'Far from showing any "resignation" to suffering and death (Jesus) seems to have opposed them with all the power at his command. He was a fighter against those elements in life which detracted from man's fullness of life, from his full health . . .'[4]

We need to observe, however, that Jesus made it quite clear that sickness was not invariably the direct consequence of sin but could be. (Compare the case of the man born blind in John 9.1-3 with the man cured at the pool of Bethzatha in John 5.1-14, especially v.14).

(v) *Jesus sometimes required faith before healing could take place, but not invariably.*
At Nazareth it is recorded 'He did not many mighty works there because of their unbelief' (Matt. 13.38). Yet clearly in the cases of the blind man of John 9, the man by the pool of Bethzatha of John 5 and the man called Legion in Mark 5, Jesus healed without being asked and demanded no conditional faith from them.

---

[1] E. G. Neal in *The Healing Power of Christ* (Hodder) p.39 makes the same observation.
[2] His article 'Disease and Healing' in the *New Bible Dictionary* (IVF 1962) p.316.
[3] See A. P. Waterson, *ibid.* p.313.
[4] *Op. cit.* p.275.

MIRACULOUS HEALING IN THE BIBLE

(vi) *Jesus's purpose in healing was primarily theological rather than philanthropic and compassionate.*
Three main factors seem to have influenced Jesus's power to perform healing miracles.

(a) He was tempted by Satan to use his miraculous powers to get a following by, for example, throwing himself from the pinacle of the temple. Jesus denounced the suggestion. Yet undoubtedly his healing miracles did create a great following. His normal injunction that those he cured should not publish the fact would apparently be the way he did not give in to the devil's temptation. But why did he persist in healing at all?

(b) We are frequently told he had compassion on the people and in about four texts this leads to miraculous healings (Matthew 14.14, 20.34, Mark 5.19, Luke 7.13).[1]

(c) By far the greatest reason for his miracles of healing were to reveal to Israel that he was none other than the Messiah whom their scriptures foretold. This point was made in various ways. When John the Baptist sent disciples to obtain confirmation of whether or not he was the expected Messiah, Jesus immediately cured many people of diseases, plague, evil spirits and blindness, and said to John's disciples, 'Go and tell John what you have seen and heard: the blind receive their sight, the lame walk, lepers are cleansed, and the deaf hear, the dead are raised up,' words which would remind John of Messianic passages of the prophet Isaiah (29.18-19, 35.5-6). Similar Messianic links can be found in Matthew 8.17 with Isaiah 53.4 and Luke 4.16-21 with Isaiah 61.1.

The fourth gospel makes the same point by referring to acts of healing as signs of who Jesus was (John 4.53-4 and 20.30-31). It also quotes Jesus as saying that his works were unique.[2]

A further illustration may also be taken from the way in which Jesus used his ability to heal as outward evidence that he had 'power on earth to forgive sins' (Matt. 9.2-7). In other words the primary purpose of the healing was to reveal who Jesus was and that he had the authority to forgive the man's sins— ultimately of greater importance than the healing of his body. However, as we shall be considering later, moral health can directly affect physical health.

Perhaps a passage in Mark 1.37-39 makes the point as conclusively as anything already written. Everyone was searching for Jesus because of the highly successful *healing* campaign he had been conducting in Galilee. However on being informed of the fact he replied: 'Let us go on to the next town that I may *preach* there also; for that is why I came out.'

[1] I have omitted Mark 1.41 as in this case there is the variant reading recording no compassion, but rather anger.
[2] See John 15.24 and the comment on it by Dr. Leon Morris in *'The Gospel according to John,'* (New London Commentaries MMS), including the 'Additional note 9: Miracles', pp.680-1 and 684-91.

(3) The Apostolic Church

The Acts of the Apostles relates quite a variety of miracles of healing such as the curing of the lame man in Acts 3, and paralytic in Acts 9.33-34. 'Extraordinary miracles' were done by means of the Apostle Paul's clothing in Acts 19.11-12. The dead were raised and evil spirits exorcized.

However that is not the whole picture. Trophimus was left behind in Miletus sick and the Apostle Paul apparently made no attempt to cure him or tried and failed (2 Tim. 4.20). Epaphroditus (Phil. 2.25-30) was critically ill and though the implication is that he temporarily recovered, it does not seem to have been by a miracle. Timothy was frequently ill, expecially with gastric trouble, but Paul prescribed a little wine (taken medicinally of course!), rather than prayer, though he may have assumed his child in the faith would have included that as well.

No-one seems sure what Paul's thorn in the flesh was, but whatever its identity Paul was not cured of it. The only other place where healing is specifically mentioned in the New Testament comes in the list of spiritual gifts in 1 Cor. 12.9, 28, 30 and James 5.14 to which I will refer again later.[1] The very absence of further reference, taken together with the failures to heal just mentioned, seems to suggest that miraculous healing was not as common a feature of the New Testament Church as is sometimes suggested. But then if miracles of healing were intended to be regular features of the Church's ministry they could hardly be called signs or extraordinary miracles. Signs and miracles, whether they refer to healing or not, are surely, almost by definition, neither frequent nor continuous? Those that occur in the Bible seem to be there for a very special purpose, namely to authenticate the special ministries of Moses, the prophets, Jesus the Messiah and the Apostles of the early Church.

The Bible teaches conclusively that God is utterly good and compassionate but that does not mean that complete healing from all bodily ailments in this life is our Christian birthright. Francis MacNutt in his most helpful book, *Healing,* to which I have referred earlier and shall refer again, makes it abundantly clear that God is more concerned for our health than for the therapeutic value of our suffering.

Nevertheless suffering is clearly within the permitted will of God in this life. God not only allowed Job to suffer but a whole host of Old Testament saints endured terrible trouble and torture (Psalm 22, Heb. 11.35-38). Ananias was specifically told that the Apostle Paul would suffer much for the sake of Christ (Acts 9.16), a prophecy amply illustrated in 2 Cor. 11 and 12 recounting Paul's beatings, stoning, shipwreck exposure, quite apart from his thorn in the flesh. In this world Jesus assured us we would have tribulation; the letters of Paul and Peter speak frequently of a suffering Church[2]; and one of the special features of the heavenly city is that it will be a place where there is no more mourning nor crying nor pain (Rev. 21.4).

C. S. Lewis devotes a helpful chapter to human pain in his famous book *The Problem of Pain.* Pain is God's megaphone to the ungodly. God uses it to shatter man's self-sufficiency so that he may be led to find his true happiness in God himself. Self-surrender to the divine will must involve

---

[1] There is no specific mention of healing in Rom. 15.19 or Heb. 2.4.
[2] See Rom. 8.18, 1 Cor. 12.26, 2 Cor. 1.6-7, Phil. 3.10, 4.12, 1 Peter 4.13.

some measure of pain, or how can man be sure he does not act from ulterior motives?'[1]

The late Malcolm Muggeridge admitted that he found suffering a mystery in a sense, but speculates on a world devoid of it, 'What a dreadful place the world would be! I would almost rather eliminate happiness. The world would be the most ghastly place because everything that corrects the tendency of this unspeakable little creature, man, to feel over important and over pleased with himself would disappear. He's bad enough now, but he would be absolutely intolerable if he never suffered.'[2]

Michael Green also speculates but from a different angle: 'How people would rush to Christianity (and for all the wrong motives) if it carried with it automatic exemption from sickness! What a nonsense it would make of Christian virtues like longsuffering, patience and endurance if instant wholeness were available for all the Christian sick! What a wrong impression it would give if salvation of physical wholeness were perfectly realised on earth whilst spiritual wholeness were partly reserved for heaven! What a very curious thing it would be if God were to decree death for all his children whilst not allowing illness for any of them!'[3]

The facts seem plain. God, as part of his very love for his creatures, sometimes uses suffering, including sickness and disease, to discipline his erring children, as could be illustrated many times from the Old Testament and specifically from Heb. 12.5-11. This is not to deny that suffering has also a *random* character—not always or necessarily related to God's disciplining of his people. 'Health is the greatest thing in the world—except sickness,' said a great saint of God. This is nothing to do with lack of real faith. Two of God's great warriors of faith in recent years have been James Hudson Taylor, founder of the China Inland Mission (now Overseas Missionary Fellowship) and George Muller, founder of the famous Bristol Orphanage, yet both were very frequently ill. Still more recently many people have been enormously helped to face the problems of life by the example of the quadriplegic Joni Eareckson.[4]

Several people famed for speaking and writing on the subject of healing in recent years have been quite seriously ill over an extended period. Mrs. Emily Gardiner Neal, author of *The Healing Power of Christ* has exercised an extensive ministry of healing in America, yet admits that for a period of nearly six years she was never for a day without pain following a spinal injury suffered in 1965 (p.xi).

The promises of total freedom from disease and suffering lie beyond this life (Rom. 8.18-23) and those who attempt to prove from Scripture that we have a right to expect full health now make the same mistake as those who attempt to teach that we should experience sinless perfection now.[5]

1 The points are all expanded by Lewis in *The Problem of Pain* (Fontana Religious paperback), pp.77-97.
2 Malcolm Muggeridge in *Jesus Rediscovered* (Collins-Fontana 1969) pp.188-9.
3 *I Believe in the Holy Spirit* (Hodder 1975) p.176.
4 See *A Further Step* by Joni Eareckson and Steve Estes, revised edition (Grand Rapids: Zondervan, 1980).
5 If Isaiah 53.4-5 refers to our sicknesses as well as it obviously does to our sins, and I understand that the original Hebrew implies that it does, I see no reason why the complete fulfilment of the prophecy must apply to this age.

3. MIRACULOUS HEALING TODAY

In the previous chapter we have sought to show that in certain stages of God's revelation of himself to men that he permitted miracles to occur and many of these were miracles of healing. Some claim that we should expect similar miracles today and that is in fact the teaching of Scripture. On what grounds do they make such claims? Let us look briefly at three:

(1) That the purpose of Christ's coming was to destroy the works of the devil (1 John 3.8a). Now no-one would dispute that this is his purpose and undoubtedly he was seen doing it during his earthly ministry. Further it is the sure and glorious promise of Scripture that he will be utterly and totally successful at the end of the age (1 Cor. 15.24-26). But the text does not in any way prove that these works of the devil, which will include sin, error, disease and death, are all being destroyed now. To suggest so seems to anticipate the end of the age.[1]

(2) Jesus Christ is the same yesterday, today and for ever (Heb. 13.8) and therefore his miraculous ministry of New Testament days should be continuing now for he never changes. But we must ask in what sense Jesus is the same. He does not wear the same body as when he was on earth. He does not live in the same place nor does he exercise the same ministry, for since his earthly ministry he has died, risen, been glorified, and now sits at the right hand of his Father interceeding for us and waiting till his enemies become his footstool. Obviously in his divine human person and character he is the same and so is the effectiveness of his redeeming work on the Cross. But to say his ministry is the same, and should be seen to be operating through his Church, then logically it should be the same in extent, method and character. That means there should be no limit to what the Church is capable of doing, healing the blind, deaf and dumb; repairing severed limbs (cf Malchus), raising the dead. Indeed why should our ministry be limited to healing alone, for Jesus walked on water, fed 5,000 from five loaves and a couple of fish, stilled storms and so on? Admittedly Jesus promised that his followers would do 'greater works' (John 14.12), but there is no indication that he had miracles of healing in mind. If he did, then there is no evidence in the New Testament that greater works of healing *were* performed than he did himself. The greater works are much more likely to refer to the preaching of the Gospel, for since Pentecost the Church has had a much wider ministry than its Master.

Further, all his healings were miraculous without recourse to any medical means or the natural recuperative powers of the human body. So those who believe in precisely the same miraculous healing ministry today as Jesus exercised on earth must be logical and renounce the use of medical, surgical and psychological means of healing. This will mean disposing of spectacles, false teeth, hearing aids, emptying the medicine cabinet and bringing all men's ills to Jesus alone. The healings will also be the same in character which will mean instantaneous, complete and permanent. But my understanding of the claims is that the healings are almost without exception gradual.

[1] The late John P. Baker attempted to argue in his small book *Salvation and Wholeness* (Fountain Trust, 1973) pp.47-8 that the church ought to be raising the dead back to life, but he seems to me substantially to weaken his case when he has to admit he has never yet personally witnessed such a raising.

MIRACULOUS HEALING TODAY

(3) The commission of Jesus provides the third answer. The contention is that the Lord commanded the disciples to go forth and heal: Matt. 10.8 'Heal the sick' and this commission similarly applies to disciples of today. But can it really possibly do so? We must take that commission in its context and there Jesus strictly told his disciples, 'Go nowhere among the Gentiles, and enter no town of the Samaritans, but go rather to the lost sheep of the house of Israel.' He also lays down a great number of other conditions that bear very little relationship to our present times, and includes in his charge that the dead shall be raised. Surely, therefore, the commission that applies to us today is that given after Jesus' resurrection in Matt. 28.18-20 where the emphasis is more on the proclamation of the Gospel, making disciples, baptizing and teaching, and there is no reference to healing. Admittedly, in the disputed ending to Mark's Gospel (Mark 16.9-10) healing is mentioned as a sign following the Gospel, and this was fulfilled in the Acts, but the actual commission was 'Go into the world and preach the Gospel to the whole creation'.[1]

If then we are given no encouragement to expect the sort of miraculous healings to-day that we associate with the ministry of Jesus, how do we account for healings that bear the marks of the miraculous?

(a) *Medically*
The British Medical Association's Committee's Report *Divine Healing and co-operation between Doctors and Clergy* lists a number of factors which complicate enquiries concerning reported 'faith-healings'. For example there can be temporary alleviations of pain and freedom from usual symptoms caused by hypnotic suggestion. 'Remissions' in the progress of certain nervous diseases, tuberculosis, leukaemia etc. are phenomena well-known to the profession, as well as 'spontaneous' cures. There are perfectly accepted medical reasons why healings may have taken place and which could equally have occurred without any outward religious actions such as prayer, or anointing or laying on of hands.

Sometimes healings have occurred for perfectly natural reasons at the same time as sacramental activities have been administered. It may seem churlish to question whether a miracle had taken place, but in all honesty it needs to be pointed out that the miracle was not in the healing process but in the timing. It could reasonably be compared with the parting of the Red Sea in Exodus 14 which has a perfectly natural and scientific explanation, but the fact that it occurred at the precise moment that the Children of Israel needed to cross was of the nature of a miracle. That is no reason why God should not be thanked.

(b) *Satanically*
I have already referred to the magicians of Egypt and their ability to do remarkable things (Exodus 7). The New Testament also narrates remarkable activities of those not motivated by the Spirit of Christ.[2]

---

[1] *Dedication* for May/June 1973 reported a case of two men who deliberately drank a potent mixture of strychnine and water. They were apparently convinced, on the basis of Mark 16.18, that they would suffer no ill-effects. Outside the Church after the service the two men doubled up in an agony of convulsive twitching—and by morning both were dead.

[2] e.g. Matt. 7.21-3, 24.24, Acts 8.9-11, 2 Thess. 2.9, 1 Tim. 4.1.

Spiritualists heal too. We are told in Scripture that the devil can appear as an 'angel of light' (2 Cor. 11.14). We need, therefore, to test the spirit according to 1 John 4 and not assume that what on the surface appears to be a miracle is therefore automatically the beneficient work of God in response to the prayer of his people.[1]

(c) *Miraculously*
In spite of all I have said there do seem to be some healings that have no other explanation, except that God in his sovereignty has intervened in an *exceptional* way. H. W. Frost gives a number of examples in his *Miraculous Healing*. The famous story of the cure of Dorothy Kerin is very well authenticated. The late Martyn Lloyd-Jones (an M.D. and M.R.C.P.) cites a number of examples in his booklet *The Supernatural in Medicine*.[2]

By now it should be apparent to my readers that if miracles happen today I believe them to be somewhat rarer than some people would have us expect. I think it very essential that we should come to this conclusion for two highly important reasons:

(1) Because I believe this is the general picture we are given in Scripture of God. He is the Creator God who is not always working miracles but has chosen to work in and through the natural order which he created and set in motion.[3] This means that generally speaking the healing of our bodies will take place by the natural processes which God has ordained: in the natural recuperative powers of the human body, in the production of antibodies to repel infection, in the formation of blood-components and the uniting of bone tissue. These are all divine processes and they will be aided by all the marvels of modern science and all the medicines and drugs that God has provided in the world he has created for our benefit.

(2) All the time some Christians are looking for God to perform miracles as soon as they are ill, they are in danger of getting depressed and disillusioned because they will feel that God has let them down because he does not act in that way. However, once they have been weaned from that false view of God, they will be in a better position to enjoy the ministry of Christian Healing that is available.

An illustration may be helpful before moving on to the practice of Christian Healing today. Jesus is recorded in Scripture as miraculously turning water into wine and feeding 5,000 with five loaves of bread and two small fishes. Yet I have not heard of Christian wine-producers, bakers and fishmongers depending *solely* on prayer for the promotion of their industries just because of the miracles of Jesus and because workers of miracles are mentioned in 1 Cor. 12.[4] Why should Christians expect to by-pass God's normal way of working when it comes to healing?

There is written up in the Ecole de Medecine in Paris the phrase 'I dressed the wound and God healed it'. I believe that from Scripture and experience that is still the normal way in which we should expect God to work today and clergy do their parishioners no service to teach them otherwise.

[1] David Watson writes helpfully on this in his book *Hidden Warfare* (S.T.L. Books) chapter 3, pp.87-94.
[2] CMF Publications, first published in October 1971.
[3] Many examples could be cited, e.g. Psalm 104.
[4] Equally, Christians in famine areas are no more proof against starvation than others.

4. CHRISTIAN HEALING TODAY

In 1 Cor. 12 the Apostle Paul writes that the Holy Spirit apportions various gifts to the Church and amongst these is that of healing (1 Cor. 12.9). Some would argue that just as the gift of Apostleship has died out, so has the gift of healing. Others say that the Church has become so unspiritual that that is the reason why we do not see the healing gift being experienced much these days. This seems a particularly weak argument seeing that it was to the Church of Corinth that Paul was writing and that Church was renowned for its lack of spirituality (1 Cor. 3.1-3).

It must certainly be acknowledged that once the early Church was launched the gift of healing was not prominent. It is not mentioned in the lists in Eph. 4.11 or Rom. 12.6-8. We are given a very full description of Christian ministry in the Pastoral Epistles but healing is never mentioned. On the other hand James 5.14 encourages us to expect to see something of the healing power of God in response to the prayer of faith and anointing with oil by the local Christian leaders. What conclusions can we draw then from these observations that can be of help to us today?

First that the ministry of healing must not be divorced from the rest of the Church's work. As the Rev. A. H. Purcell Fox has written, 'We must not allow the healing ministry to be lifted out of its setting in the larger ministry of the Church, for to do so would be to let it degenerate into a cult.'[1] John Baker supports this view in an article in *The Churchman* in which he writes 'We need ... to integrate the ministry of healing and prayer for the sick into the whole ministry of the Gospel in the Church. As long as it is a separate "thing", it is bound to be out of perspective.'[2] I agree with this and therefore question special healing missions unless the salvation of the whole person is in mind. General intercessions for the sick should surely form part of supplications when the body of Christ normally gathers for prayer, whether it be for a public service on Sunday or a prayer meeting on Church premises or in a house group during the week.

Secondly, that to some people within the Church the Holy Spirit may give a special gift of healing. To possess such a gift will not necessarily mean that the holder performs miracles, but rather becomes an especial channel of God's healing love and compassion to others in partnership with the medical profession. What follows, I hope, will illustrate what I mean.

One of the most helpful books to be written on healing recently is that entitled *Healing* by the American Roman Catholic priest, Francis MacNutt O.P. He distinguishes four basic areas of sickness, each of which require its own appropriate treatment. They can be briefly summarized as follows:

(1) Moral sickness caused by our own sin.
(2) Emotional sickness caused by anxiety and emotional hurts of our past.
(3) Physical sickness caused by disease or accident.
(4) 'Spiritual' sickness caused by demonic oppression.

[1] *The Church's Ministry of Healing* (Longmans).
[2] *The Churchman* Vol. 86 No. 4 Winter 1972 p.268.

Of course I have separated these for convenience and will enlarge on each separately, but an individual who is sick may well need treatment in more than one area. For example, a person suffering from VD will need antibiotics, but also moral help.

Let us now look at these four areas and make some recommendations concerning treatment.

(1) Moral sickness

'When I declared not my sin, my body wasted away through my groaning all day long. For day and night thy hand was heavy upon me; my strength was dried up as by the heat of summer,' (Ps. 32.3-4). The Psalmist writes in the context of a psalm of a man who knows the blessings of life when he knows his sins are forgiven. (Cf. Ps. 103.2-3).

Jesus on a number of occasions told people suffering from physical sickness that their sins were forgiven (eg Matt. 9.1-8) before effecting any physical cure.

The Apostle Paul warns the Corinthian Christians to examine themselves before receiving the sacramental elements, adding 'For anyone who eats and drinks without discerning the body eats and drinks judgment upon himself. That is why many of you are weak and ill, and some have died.' (1 Cor. 11.29-30).[1]

In my ministry there are a number of people who come readily to mind whom I knew harboured an unforgiving spirit and persisted in doing so, despite much exhortation to confess. In one case it was no surprise to me that cancer developed and the person died. This does not mean, of course, that this will always be the case or that all cancer patients harbour an unforgiving spirit.

Many people in our parishes, even though professing Christians, suffer from a great many anxieties, but this is contradictory to trust in our all-loving and all-caring God. Jesus makes quite plain in the sermon on the mount that we should not worry (Matt. 6.25-34).

Years ago as a student I thought I had failed an examination and was seriously concerned about my future as a result. At the time I was also suffering from extreme pain in my right arm, not only making a temporary job almost impossible but reducing me at times to tears. The doctor examined me, X-rayed the arm, but could find nothing wrong. Then I learned that I had passed the exam, and the pain in my arm vanished.

Francis MacNutt says, 'There is good evidence, then, that there is a very natural connection between much of our sickness and our spiritual and emotional health.'[2]

In an issue of *ACE,*[3] Michael Wright writes:

> 'In my pastoral work in my parish I have found so many people who live under stress. They cannot really relax. Many cannot sleep well, they get depressed. An astonishing

---

[1] Dr. Martyn Lloyd-Jones enlarges on this very point in his exposition of Eph. 5.18-6.9, *Life in the Spirit* (Banner of Truth Trust, 1974) p.179.
[2] *Healing,* p.171.
[3] The quarterly bulletin of the Archbishops' Council on Evangelism, Diocesan House, Quarry Street, Guildford, Surrey GU1 3XG. (This publication is now discontinued).

CHRISTIAN HEALING TODAY

number are regularly taking tranquilizers. One local doctor says that half the patients who come to him come because of spiritual problems and stress.

'Their illness stems from things like a guilt feeling, bad relationships in their home life, a row with their neighbours, a feeling of being inadequate, insecure, angry, jealous, afraid, lonely, or just generally dissatisfied with life. The body's reaction to this spiritual malaise can vary from asthma, skin diseases and insomnia, to ulcers, angina, pains which come and go and cannot easily be identified.'

For those in the ministry these facts should find a place in their preaching and pastoral work. People must be brought to see that they must repent of their sins and put their personal faith in Jesus Christ as their Saviour. They must then be assured that if they really have done this that they are forgiven. However, they must also realise that this is not only an initial experience, but that day by day there is going to be the need for an earnest prayer 'Forgive us our sins as we forgive those who sin against us.'

For some this may prove very difficult and the Book of Common Prayer makes provision for it in the first exhortation in the Communion Service:

'And because it is requisite, that no man should come to the Holy Communion, but with a full trust in God's mercy, and with a quiet conscience; therefore if there be any of you, who by this means cannot quiet his own conscience herein, but requireth further comfort or counsel, let him come to me, or to some other discreet and learned Minister of God's Word, and open his grief; that by the ministry of God's holy Word he may receive the benefit of absolution, together with ghostly counsel and advice, to the quieting of his conscience, and avoiding of all scruple and doubtfulness.'

The Book of Common Prayer contains general directions and a formula for the absolution of the sick in the Order for the Visitation of the Sick.

A woman known to me had very great domestic problems and worried very deeply, so much so that she became thin and ill. After much prayer and discussion we held a short service of Holy Communion in the home of friends with whom she had received much spiritual counsel. We especially prayed that she might know the Lord's peace that passes all understanding and we corporately laid hands on her. A little while later I saw her entering heartily in the games at a New Year's party—a transformed person rejoicing in the forgiveness and peace of the Lord.

In the article in *ACE* from which I quoted previously Michael Wright describes how he and Peggy Satow organized a course of four sessions entitled 'Relax and feel better'. Forty people enrolled, ranging from social workers and hospital sisters, to shop assistants, housewives, a finance controller, librarians and school teachers. Some were members of his church, but most were not. Outlining this course he says 'We taught a simple approach to relaxed living, deep breathing exercises, relaxation, walking, sitting and laying on the floor. We taught a discipline of simple meditation, first on one word, then broadening out on to three themes: forgiveness, acceptance, communion. Our concern was to teach not just physical exercises, but a new relationship between people, and between ourselves and God, helping people to see how to apply the Two Great Commandments as a principle of life and of personal health.' Considerable further help on this aspect can be found in Jean C. Grigor *Grow to Love, A Resource Book for Groups* (The Saint Andrew Press, Edinburgh, 1977).

(2) Emotional sickness

Some people have emotional and psychological problems that go much deeper than the sort we were thinking about above. They suffer from mental depression, compulsive tendencies, irrational fears and anxieties, which they find difficult to understand and impossible to cope with. For many the kindest advice that the minister may give is to recommend a psychiatrist, preferably one who has embraced the Christian faith.

Many ministers today have also been greatly helped in dealing with such people through the insights gained from Clinical Theology[1] and from such books as *I'm OK, You're OK*.[2]

Some of these emotional problems stem from the past, even in some cases from before birth. Our task is to help bring the causes from the subconscious to the surface so that the emotionally sick person can come to terms with the problem. The psychiatrist will do this by various means such as drugs, hypnosis and dream analysis. The Christian has a further method, namely prayer. The one person who really knows the cause of the problem and has the power to release the sick person is Jesus himself.

A friend of a relative of mine was deeply troubled in her spiritual life and asked my relative to pray for her, which she was pleased to do. In her prayers she frequently became aware of a pond at the bottom of a garden, so enquired if this meant anything. 'Oh yes,' was the reply, 'my father committed suicide in the pond at the bottom of our garden.' The Lord in his gracious wisdom was bringing to the surface the deep-seated anxiety in this person's life. Mrs. Neal writes about the healing of the memories on pages 118-9 of *The Healing Power of Christ*. There are also three books on this subject included in the Bibliography on p.25 by Robert Faricy, Michael Scanlan and Ruth Carter Stapleton.

When we are seeking to help people with such problems we shall want them to feel they can confide in us without fear of what they say going further. We should obviously respect this but at the same time we do want to enlist as much prayer support from the local church as possible.

One young man with whom I had much to do and who went through agonies of depression gradually came to discover the basic causes of his trouble with the considerable assistance of a very qualified Christian counsellor. He also shared his problems with me and asked for special prayer of the congregation. Immediately following the distribution of the elements at an evening Communion Service he came to the chancel steps and I together with other 'elders' of the church laid hands on him.[3] I prayed a very explicit extempore prayer which both I and quite a number of my congregation felt was Spirit-led. It was evident to many that I could not possibly have prayed in that way had I not first had the young man's permission. There was a marked improvement in his life from that evening and he is now happily married with two children.

[1] For details write to the Director, Lingdale, Weston Avenue, Mount Hooton Road, Nottingham NG7 4BA.
[2] By Thomas A. Harris (Pan Books).
[3] I usually pray on such occasions as follows: 'A.B., receive from our Lord Jesus Christ all that he purposes to give you in the healing of your body, mind and spirit, for his glory's sake.' The response is 'I thank you, Lord.' On this occasion I departed from the usual form.

CHRISTIAN HEALING TODAY

(3) Physical sickness

In dealing with healing under this heading it would perhaps be helpful to repeat very briefly some conclusions made earlier in this booklet:

(a) That we are given no encouragement to expect miraculous healing of the kind exercised by Jesus, but that does not mean we are to expect nothing. Did not Jesus say: 'Truly, I say to you, whoever says to this mountain, "Be taken up and cast into the sea," and does not doubt in his heart, but believes that what he says will come to pass, it will be done for him. Therefore I tell you, whatever you ask in prayer, believe be done for him. Therefore I tell you, whatever you ask in prayer, believe that you receive it, and you will.' (Mk. 11.23-24).

In claiming that promise in prayer it must also not conflict with the rest of biblical teaching on prayer or healing. We are never in a position to demand a specific response, since we may never dictate to our sovereign Lord precisely how he shall act in answer to our prayers. To suggest, as some do, that this shows lack of faith is to misunderstand the relationship between God's sovereignty and man's faith. If we divorce the two 'then we will fall into the trap of thinking that if we can produce enough of it (faith) we can get God to do what we want'. Such thinking in fact turns Scripture on its head, for it ends up with a faith that God will obey us, rather than a faith which enables us to obey God. It is right to affirm that *God uses our faith*, it is blasphemy to believe that our Faith can use god—and the small 'g' is deliberate, because whatever we are able to *use* is not God with a capital 'G'![1]

(b) We should make full use of all the medical means that God has put at our disposal including medicine and the wisdom and skill of surgeons, doctors, nurses, physiotherapists, etc., who are, after all, aiming to remove all the obstacles they can which might prevent the God-given natural ability of the body and mind to heal itself.

(c) Unless Jesus returns first we shall eventually die.

What action can we take when someone is ill? Obviously we can pray, yet we are all familiar with the prayer that includes the phrase 'If it be your will, lay your healing hands on John (or Mary).' If they recover it was the Lord's will. If they don't it wasn't, and we are left feeling a bit sceptical about praying for the sick.

However, surely we shall always be open to this sort of charge about prayer on any subject, not only on healing. There is a story told of a Quaker preacher being interrupted when preaching on the subject of 'Prayer' by the remark, 'I don't believe in prayer'. 'Dost thou ever pray, friend?' the preacher enquired. 'No, not I', was the reply. 'Then what dost thou know about it, friend?' As Archbishop William Temple used to say to his sceptical enquirers about prayer: 'When I pray, coincidences happen. When I don't they don't.'

---

[1] From *Faith and Healing* by John Richards (Renewal Servicing, P.O. Box 366, Addlestone, Weybridge, Surrey KT15 3UL).

CHRISTIAN HEALING IN THE PARISH

Those of us who believe in prayer, whether for the sick or anyone else, are quite simply placing the whole situation into the hands of God, in the confidence that whatever the outcome he knows best.[1]

On a number of occasions I have had to minister for some while to people for whom the doctors had given up hope. I had not given up hope, but to be realistic believed that death should be considered a real possibility. The sick person and those closely associated with the person felt it showed lack of faith to admit such a possibility. So a charade took place in which a number of people pretended against their better judgment that the person would soon be up and about again. This had very regrettable consequences such as a sense of strain at the bedside, no opportunity to speak openly about the biblical teaching on death and heaven and no encouragement to put one's earthly affairs in order (such as making a will, etc.). And when death has occurred, as it frequently has, there has been much heart-searching by the bereaved as to where they had failed to exercise enough faith and perhaps, too, an unspoken feeling that God has somehow let them down. A keen but much troubled Christian young man said to me when a churchwarden died, to which I refer later, 'How can we believe in prayer any more?' I simply replied, 'But God has answered for we have stopped praying, knowing he is now with Jesus, which is far better.'[2]

I referred in the Preface to the death of David Watson, which was undoubtedly seen by many involved in the healing ministry as a considerable embarrassment, especially bearing in mind the volume of prayer offered world-wide for his recovery, quite apart from the variety of ministrations he received during the final year of his remarkable life as he wrestled with cancer. But despite the prophecies and other assurances of answered prayer, the one person that was closest to the truth was his medical consultant, who gave him just about a year to live from the time the trouble was located. John Richards has very helpfully considered the implications of David's death in *Way of Life* for July—September 1984 (published by the Guild of Health Ltd. at 26 Queen Anne Street, London W1M 9LB). John especially stresses that God does not decide on how he will act depending on the *quantity* or prayer offered.

The reason that I mention the matter, however, is because reading between the lines of David's book *Fear No Evil* I believe his last year on earth would have been considerably eased if only the whole situation could have confidently been placed in the hands of God and left there, recognising his physical death was a very real possibility.

By contrast the days that led up to the death of Bishop John Robinson, former Bishop of Woolwich, in December 1983 seemed so much more relaxed as outlined in Richard Harries book *Prayer and the Pursuit of Happiness* (Fount Paperbacks, London, 1985) pp.124-5.

---

[1] Mrs. E. G. Neal's book *The Healing Power of Christ* (Hodder) chapter 6 makes the same point.

[2] For further reading on this subject see *When the Spirit Comes* (Hodder) pp.115-123 in which the author, Colin Urquhart, describes the death of 'Gomer' and the lessons learnt from it. See also E. G. Neal *The Healing Power of Christ* (Hodder), chapter 2.

Perhaps the most helpful illustration I know on this vital issue of committing our sickness into the hands of God and accepting his sovereign will comes the pen of Catherine Marshall in her book *Beyond Ourselves*[1]:

> 'One afternoon a pamphlet was put in my hand. It was the story of a missionary who had been an invalid for eight years. Constantly she had prayed that God would make her well, so that she might do his work. Finally, worn out with futile petition she prayed, "All right, I give up. If you want me to be an invalid for the rest of my days, that's your Business. Anyway, I've discovered that I want you more even than I want my health. You decide." The pamphlet said that within two weeks the woman was out of bed, completely well.
>
> 'This made no sense to me. It seemed too pat. Yet I could not forget the story. On the morning of September 14th I came to the same point of abject acceptance. "I'm tired of asking" was the burden of my prayer. "I'm beaten, finished. God, you decide what you want for me for the rest of my life . . ." Tears flowed. I had no faith as I understood faith. I expected nothing. The gift of my sick self was made with no trace of graciousness.
>
> 'The result was as if windows had opened in heaven; as if some dynamo of heavenly power had begun flowing, flowing into me. From that moment my recovery began.'

We must also include the sick in our general Church intercessions.

The young daughter of a curate of mine had spinal trouble which doctors seemed unable to diagnose. She was admitted to hospital where she remained for some months. But prayer was offered up almost daily by the parish. Meanwhile I asked my curate to do most of the sick visiting in that hospital and I would visit parishioners in the other hospitals in the area. Suddenly the curate's child, for no apparent reason and to the doctors' astonishment, recovered. Later however her father was appointed official Chaplain to the hospital and subsequently to several other hospitals in the area and has continued to be for over 23 years. Had there been a purpose behind her illness?

Sometimes it may be appropriate to combine prayer with laying-on-of-hands. An elderly lady and very keen Christian was having considerable trouble with her breathing which was causing her especial trouble at night. Friends gathered at her house for a short Communion Service. I read from Phil. 1.19-24 and explained that the Apostle Paul was of a divided mind. On the one hand he wanted to die and be more intimately with Christ. On the other hand to remain alive meant further fruitful labour on earth. The same possibilities lay before this radiant Christian woman. We did not know which was the Lord's will for her. After receiving Communion we all gathered round and laid hands on her. I prayed that either the Lord would take her quickly to be with him or her breathing problem would cease. It did and she was soon back worshipping with us in church.

A young boy from a Christian home had been having blackouts, was off his food and generally very poorly. Without warning I just dropped in on my own and in as unpretentious way as possible we talked about the love of Jesus for children and how he obviously enjoyed seeing them out playing games. Apparently casually I asked the boy if he would like me to

[1] Published by Peter Davies (London) pp.93-4.

talk to Jesus about his trouble, which we did. As far as one could see his health steadily improved from that day and he told his mother he was glad I had called.

In the case of very serious illness I believe we should minister to the sick in accordance with James 5.14-15. What can we say about this passage?

(i) It is clear that the sick person is sufficiently unwell to be housebound, probably confined to bed.
(ii) Prayer is to be offered.
(iii) Oil is to be used. This was used medically in biblical times and is sacramentally associated with the Holy Spirit who also is responsible for distributing gifts of healing (1 Cor. 12.9).
(iv) The word 'save' and 'raise up' are precisely the words used for salvation on the one hand and the resurrection on the other. So when we pray such a prayer we can be absolutely confident that it is going to be answered, but we cannot tell whether it will be in this life or in the life to come. For the Christian the latter is in fact far better, for it is only there that all the limitations and frustrations and infirmities of this mortal life will be transformed. (See Rom. 8.22-23, 1 Cor. 2.9, 15.42-57, 2 Cor. 4.16-5.5, Rev. 21.1-4).

I once held a service of anointing at the hospital bedside for a much-loved and well-known churchwarden who had cancer. Prayers were being offered up for him in various parts of the country. He was greatly uplifted by the service but was physically dead in three weeks.

More recently a number of us gathered in a home of a woman who had been deeply depressed and possibly suffering from some blood deficiency. The doctors had her in hospital and applied tests to no avail. We read James 5 noting the various points made above. We planned no formal service but had a period of extempore prayer. I then anointed the woman with oil and prayed a prayer based on James 5. Within a few weeks the woman was admitting to my wife after church that she had not felt so much better for a long time. She was soon back at work and her blood condition was improving. She still occasionally has poorly turns and both the medical profession and the church continue to minister to her.

Of course very seriously ill patients are not necessarily house-bound, so there does not seem to be any particular reason why anointing should only be restricted to them.

Some people believe that the 'prayer of faith' referred to by James and the 'faith' mentioned by Jesus in Mark 11.22-23 is a 'given' faith. The late Dr. Martyn Lloyd-Jones wrote of it: *'No one can work it up:* he either has it or he does not have such faith. It partly depends upon a man's general spirituality and his general faith in God, *and still more upon his sovereign will.'*[1] A clergyman friend of mine was billed to speak on the subject of Healing at his Church meeting, but when the day came he had such a bad cold he was confined to bed. He did not relish the prospect of a further notice across the one advertising the meeting 'Lecture postponed—Rector ill'! However, the Lord gave him a special gift 'of faith' and he recovered in time to give his talk.

[1] *The Supernatural in Medicine* (CMF Publications) p.22. (The italics are mine).

Since the original edition of this booklet was published several booklets have appeared relating to liturgical services for the sick, namely my own *Pastoral and Liturgical Ministry to the Sick* (Grove Booklet on Ministry and Worship no. 59, 1978), *Ministry to the Sick* (Authorized Alternative Services) and *Liturgy for the Sick: The New Church of England Services* by Colin Buchanan and David Wheaton (Grove Worship Series no. 84, 1983). Further information on this subject can also be obtained from the Guild of St. Raphael, St. Paul's House, 77 Kirmston Street, London SW1. For a much more detailed study readers are referred to Professor Gusmer's book listed in the bibliography.

If it seems appropriate to pray, lay on hands or anoint within the context of Holy Communion then an abbreviated rite that is familiar and preferred by the patient should obviously be the overriding factor.

(4) 'Spiritual' sickness caused by demonic oppression

This whole subject came into particular prominence some years ago through a widely reported incident in South Yorkshire. A word or two here will be appropriate.

The following guidelines on Exorcism were given by the Archbishop of Canterbury on 30 June 1975:

> 'The Christian ministry is a ministry of deliverance and healing. Jesus Christ exercised such a ministry and has commended its continuance to his church.
> There are many men and women so within the grip of the power of evil that they need the aid of the Christian Church in delivering them from it. When this ministry is carried out the following factors should be borne in mind:
> 1. It should be done in collaboration with the resources of medicine.
> 2. It should be done in the context of prayer and sacrament.
> 3. It should be done with a minimum of publicity.
> 4. It should be done by experienced persons authorized by the Diocesan Bishop.
> 5. It should be followed up by continuing pastoral care.
>
> The Bishops are continuing to keep these issues under review in order to be of maximum help to those who seek their guidance.'

I could name a number of people who have been very greatly helped by a ministry of exorcism. One girl, a student at Leeds University, stands out vividly in my memory. She had been deeply involved in the occult from childhood and was the slave of some evil presence when I first met her. She dressed totally in black with dark make-up, especially around the eyes. She had been confirmed as a child—part of the school routine, I believe. Several Christian students known to the girl and some of my staff gathered for a simple Communion Service and deliverance ministry, for which I obtained permission from one of my bishops. At the point where I rebuked the evil spirit and demanded in the name of Jesus Christ that it leave her she fell to the ground, writhing. People quoted appropriate scriptural texts and encouragement. Slowly but surely she rose from the ground smiling and expressed surprise at how bright the colours were in the small chapel. She was in church the following Sunday, brightly dressed, accompanied by several students amazed at the change in her life. She handed me a card expressing her appreciation for the church's ministry. John Richards, author of the book *But Deliver us from Evil*[1] has written Grove Booklet no. 44 on the subject entitled *Exorcism, Deliverance and Healing: Some Pastoral Guidelines* published in May 1976. I commend it to my readers.

[1] Darton, Longman & Todd 1974. Mr. Richards has been secretary of the Bishop of Exeter's Study Group on Exorcism.

5. CONCLUSION

Obviously in a booklet of this size one cannot deal with so vast a subject anything like adequately and I commend the bibliography to those who want to study the matter further. My aim has been to face the facts of life, sickness and death, squarely and openly, but with the supreme optimism of the Apostle Paul who wrote 'in all things we are more than conquerors through him who loved us.' The Apostle goes on to say: 'I am sure that neither death, nor life, nor angels, nor principalities, nor things present, nor things to come, nor powers, nor height, nor depth, nor anything else in all creation, will be able to separate us from the love of God in Christ Jesus our Lord' (Rom. 8.37-39).

I am convinced that there should be a ministry of Christian Healing in our parishes and I hope I may have encouraged other ordinary and busy Christians like myself to come to the same conclusion. If I have given the impression in places that I have mainly written for clergy, that is not intentional, for I believe the ministry of healing should be exercised by the whole church. However I think we have to face the fact that in most parochial situations it is still true that the pastor is expected to give the lead if there are to be any changes in attitudes or administration. May we all, clergy and laity together, discover to the full all that 'the Lord our Healer' has promised us. (Exodus 15.26).

Jesus Christ as part of his full sharing of our humanity experienced the need for sleep, food and drink, etc. Yet I believe he was the one person born into the world who enjoyed perfect physical, mental and spiritual health. (Some people confused need for sleep etc. with illness). This health he abandoned when he quite deliberately bore our sins and carried our sicknesses on the Cross.

That very act has guaranteed for all those that love him eventual perfect wholeness—in heaven. Meanwhile on this side of the grave our 'knowledge is imperfect . . . Now we see in a mirror dimly, but then face to face. Now I know in part, then I shall understand fully.' (1 Cor. 13.9, 12). Or in the words of one who suffered much in his lifetime, William Cowper:

> 'Blind unbelief is sure to err,
> And scan his work in vain.
> God is his own interpreter,
> And he will make it plain.'

Detached footnote (see footnote on p.6 above):

A widely-known American Episcopalian recounted to a gathering of clergy in St. Alban's Diocesan House in July 1973 of a woman whose leg was completely and instantaneously healed of a severe fracture following a simple prayer for relief from pain. Prior to the healing the leg was actually two inches shorter. A friend of mine present in the meeting followed the story up. After considerable correspondence a letter from the woman's own doctor included the following statement: '. . . she had multiple fractures of the pelvis which eventually healed in good position. She had X-rays of her extremities at the time of this accident but no evidence of any fracture involving the long bones of the lower extremities. My records do not reflect any shortening of either extremity and no fractures of the extremities, so I cannot give you any further information as to the nature of the complaint which apparently cleared up "miraculously".'